Herbs That Cure

Anaemia

Time-Tested Herbal Remedies

No Side-effects

by

Prayank

Contents

Rose for..

Saunf for..

Turmeric for..

Vasaka for..

Some Important Notes

Introduction

Anemia is the most common disorder of the blood. Anemia symptoms can be minor or vague. Most commonly, people with anemia report a feeling of weakness, or fatigue, general malaise and sometimes poor concentration. They may also report shortness of breath. In very severe anemia, the patient may have palpitations, angina (if heart disease is also present), intermittent claudication of the legs, and symptoms of heart failure.

In the book, you will find brief details of herbs and some common food items that help you cure anaemia. It also gives you an option to choose what is easily available in your locality. Herb names may be different in different places, hence you should rely on botanical names to find how it is known in a particular place/location.

Though there are people who treat ailments inexpensively with herbal remedies, most consider it as the last minute miracle worker once all other avenues of treatments have been exhausted.

Such an approach discounts the sophisticated and elaborately documented information dealing with specific medicinal applications of herbs for specific complaints. These methods of herbal remedies are designed for optimum beneficial use and tested innumerable times in actual practice.

Almond

(Pranus amygdalus)

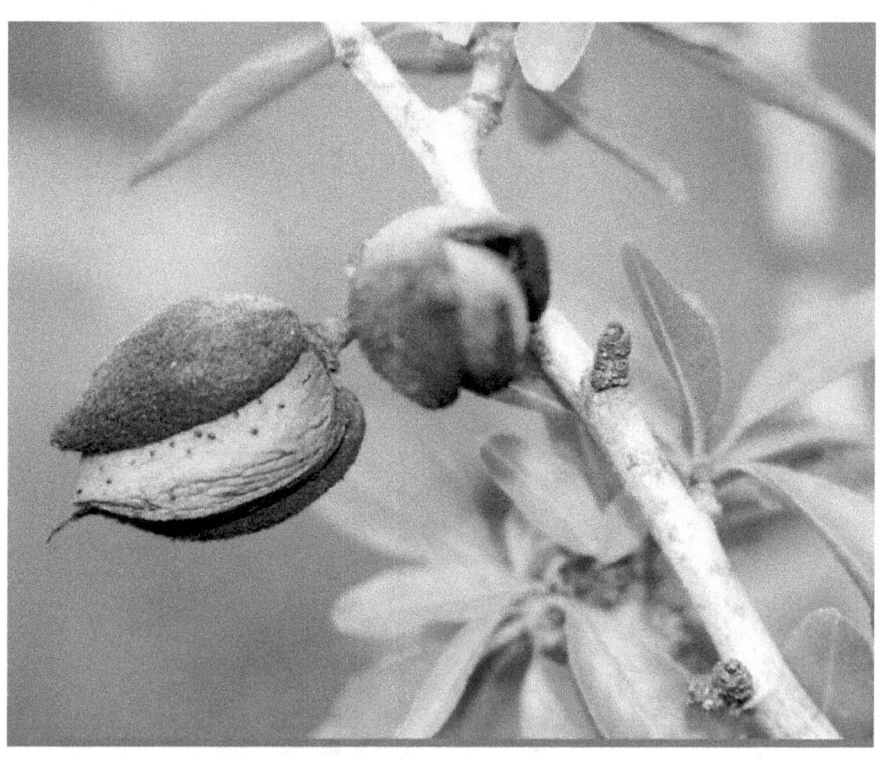

General

Almond contains twenty percent protein – a percentage one finds hardly anywhere else in the plant kingdom. Moreover, the quality of protein is such that it is easily digested. It is considered to be an ideal supplement to milk.

Profile

Botanical Name : Pranus dulcis, Pranus amygdalus, Pranus communis, Amygdalus communis

Family :

Appearance : A tree growing to the height of around 9 meters.

Medicinal Parts : Kernel, oil, shell

Distribution : The almond is native to the Mediterranean region of the Middle East, eastward as far as the Indus. It was spread by humans in ancient times along the shores of the Mediterranean into northern Africa and southern Europe and more recently transported to other parts of the world, notably California, United States.

Preparation and Dose

Soak 8-10 almonds and 1 tsp rice overnight. Remove the outer skin of almond. Grind into fine paste. Mix in some milk and a pinch of turmeric powder. Boil and drink along with sugar candy for taste.

<u>Caution</u> : The brown outer skin of almond causes excessive heat in the body, so it should be consumed after removing this skin during summer months and in hot climatic zones.

Banana

(Musa paradisiaca)

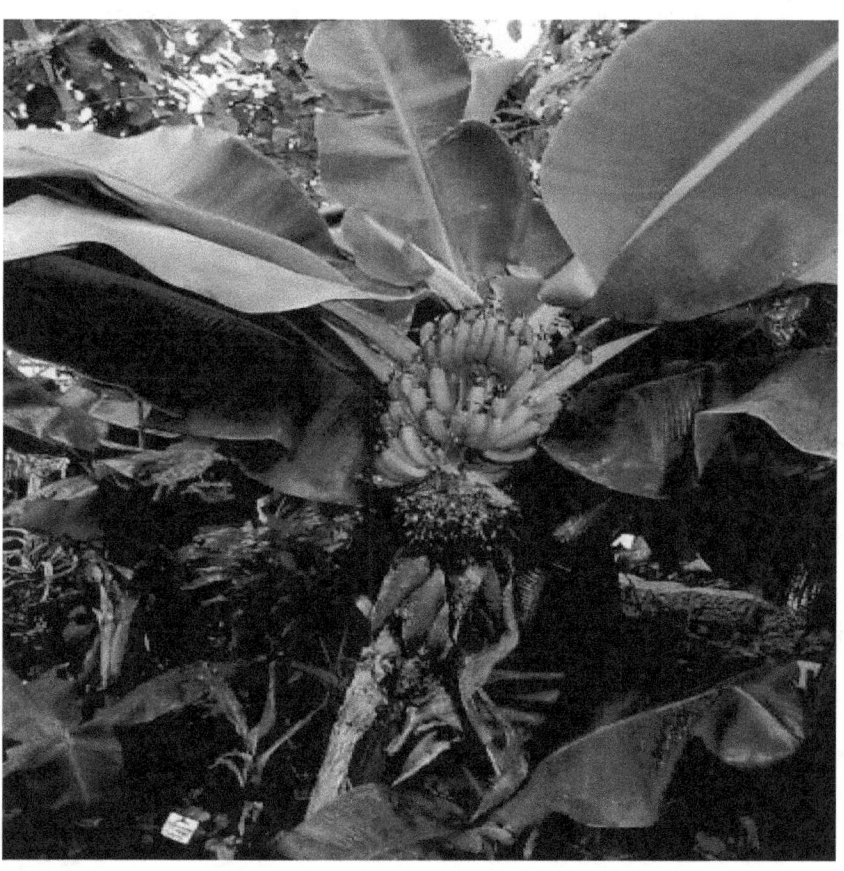

General

The term "banana" is used as the common name for the plants which produce the fruit, and the fruit itself. Fruits (unripe or ripe) and the edible rootstock have several curative properties.

Profile

Botanical Name : Musa paradisiaca, Musa sapientuum

Family : Musaceau

Appearance : A tall herb with aerial pseudo stem, dying after flowering. Leaves – large, oblong, narrowed to base. Flowers – in spikes, drooping with conspicuous bracts, dull brown. Fruits – in several clusters, generally golden yellow on ripening.

Medicinal Parts : Root, stem, sheath, leaves, flower, fruits.

Distribution : Native to tropical South and Southeast Asia, they are now grown in at least 107 countries, primarily for their fruit, and to a lesser extent to make fiber, banana wine and as ornamental plants.

Preparation and Dose

- Take a ripe banana along with 1 tsp honey. Or,

- Mix 1 tbsp juice of amla with a ripe, mashed banana. Eat 2-3 times a day. Or,

- Burn some of the root in fire. Collect the ash. Take ¼ tsp of this ash mixed with honey for a few days.

Carrots

(Daucus carota)

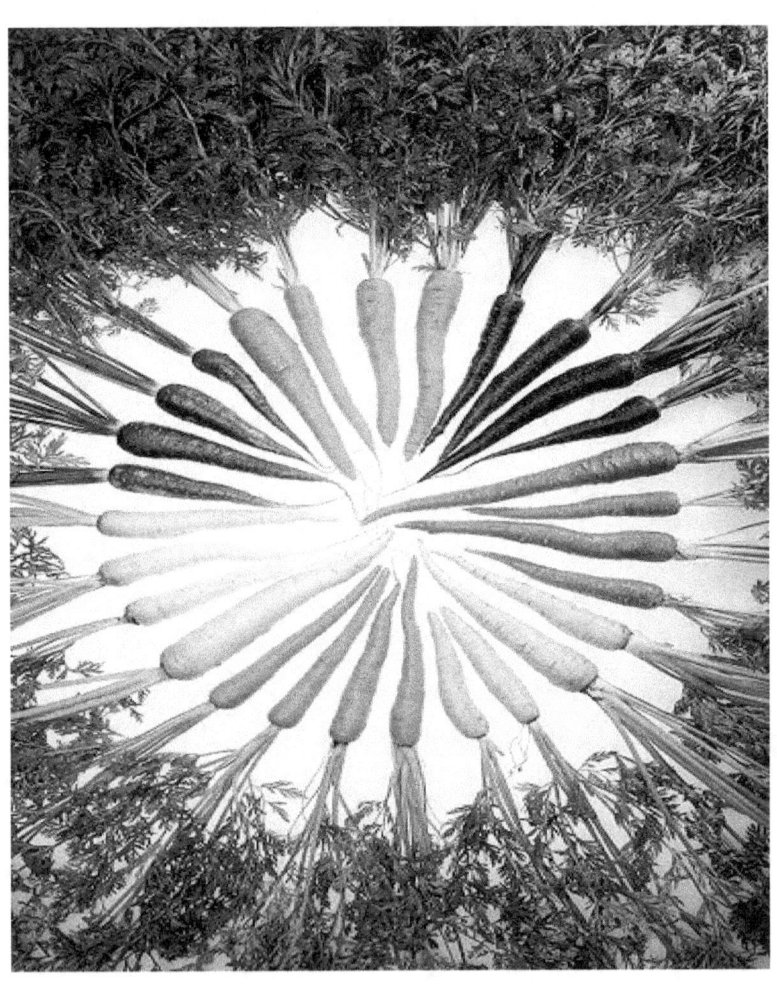

General

This common yet popular tuber can be eaten both raw and cooked. It contains good amounts of Vitamins - A, B and C besides starch, sugar, iron, calcium and phosphorous.

Profile

Botanical Name : Daucus carota

Other Species : Bee's nest, wild carrot

Family : Umbelliferae

Appearance : An annual or biennial herb. Stem - hairy and branched. Leaves - in fine divisions. Flowers - lacy white in clusters.

Medicinal Parts : Root(cultivated), leaves, seeds(wild)

Distribution : Generally available in most parts of world.

Preparation and Dose

Frequent intake of carrot juice is beneficial in case of anaemia.

Mix 2 tbsp of honey in a cup of carrot juice and drink for few weeks.

Drink 1 to 2 cups of juice in a day.

Cinnamon

(Cinnamomum zeylanicum)

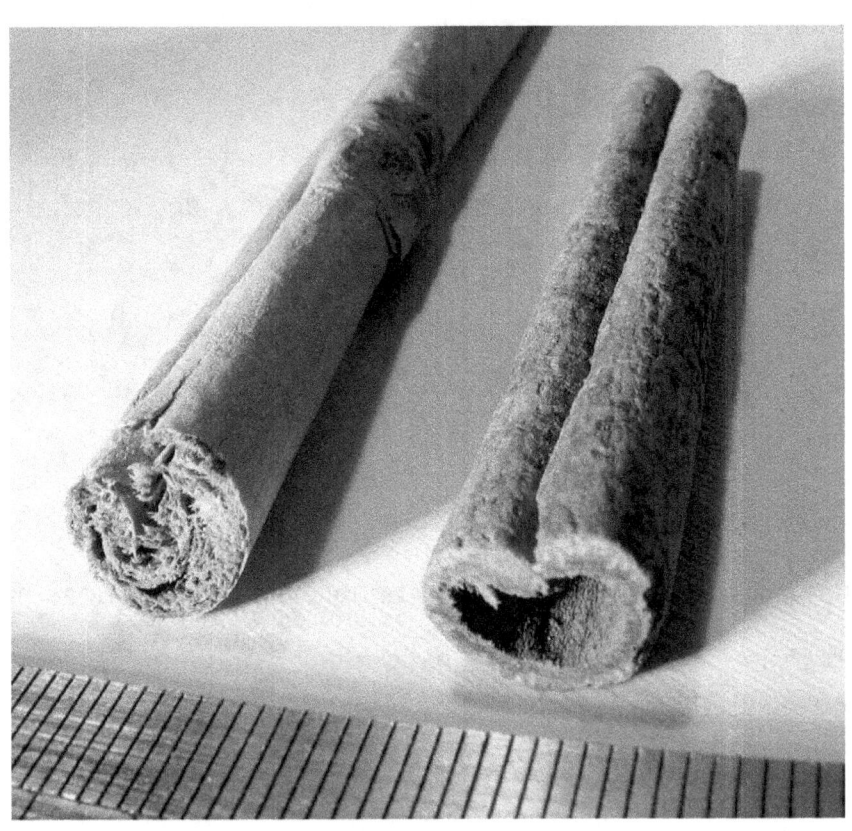

General

The stem bark which is commonly used as a flavoring agent also possesses medicinal properties. Cinnamon strengthens the heart, stimulates the kidneys, fights toxins, and harmonizes the flow of circulation.

Profile

Botanical Name : Cinnamomum zeylanicum, Cinnamomum verum

Family : Lauraceae

Appearance : Evergreen tree with large, leathery leaves and minute flowers in hairy clusters.

Medicinal Parts : bark of the stem and oil from it.

Distribution : SriLanka produces 80-90% of the world's supply of Cinnamomum verum, and this species is also cultivated on a commercial scale in Seychelles and Madagascar. Global production of the other species comes from Indonesia (produces around two-thirds of the total), with significant production in China. India and Vietnam are also minor producers.

Preparation and Dose

Dissolve powdered cinnamon (1 tsp) and 2 tsp honey in 2 cups pomegranate juice. Dosage – ½ cup.

Coriander

(Coriandrum sativum)

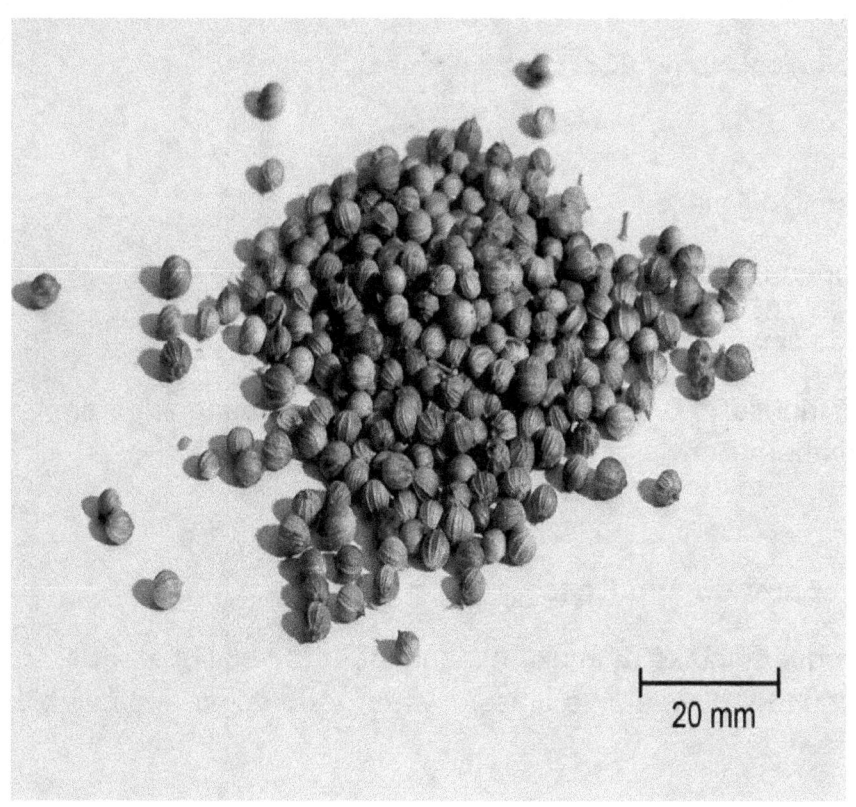

20 mm

General

Coriander (Coriandrum sativum), also known as cilantro, Chinese parsley or dhania is an annual herb, well known for its carminative and cooling properties. Both leaves of coriander and its seeds are effective household remedy for many ailments.

Profile

Botanical Name : Coriandrum sativum

Family : Apiaceae

Appearance : Aromatic herb with dissected leaves.

Medicinal Parts : Leaves, seeds

Distribution : Coriander is native to regions spanning from southern Europe and North Africa to southwestern Asia.

Preparation and Dose

Frequent intake of intake of coriander tea : boil or steep 2 tsp coriander powder in a glass of water. Add sugar and milk to taste.

Dronapushpi

(Leucas Aspera)

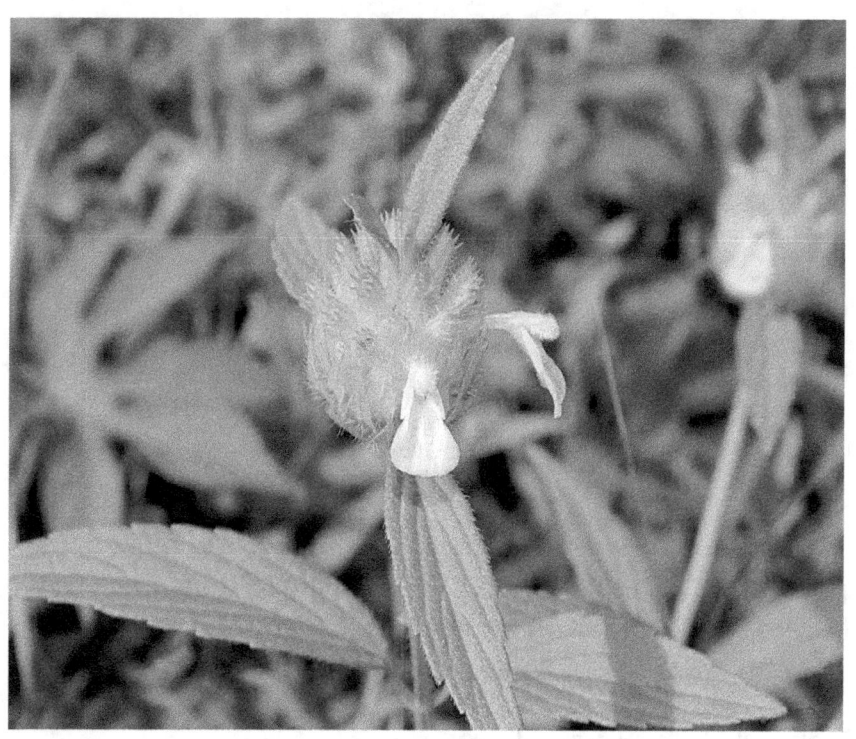

General

Like many other medicinal plants, Dronapushpi grows in wilderness and in wastelands. The flowering annual herb is a common weed which also has uses as an edible vegetable and herbal remedy. It has many common names, including guma, dronpushpi or drona puspi, and tou xu bai rong cao. It is a common plant across Asia from China to the Indian subcontinent.

It springs up in cultivated fields as a weed, especially after a period of rain and is readily available in markets. One of the plant's most common historical uses has been as a treatment for snakebite

Profile

Botanical Name : Leucas aspera

Other Species : leucas cephalotes

Family : Lamiaceae

Appearance : Erect herb, 1-2 ft tall with single opposite leaves. Flowers- white, small, in axiles. Corola -2 lipped, upper lip short and hairy, lower lip twice as long.

Medicinal Parts : Leaf, Flower

Distribution : Found in India, Bangladesh, Mauritius, and in several SE Asian countries.

Preparation

Grind equal quantities of leaves of Dronapushpi, Keezhanelli and Karisilanganni into a very fine paste.

(Keezhanelli and Karisilanganni – brief profiles given below)

Dose

Take 1 tbsp of paste with buttermilk in the morning hours.

Keezhanelli

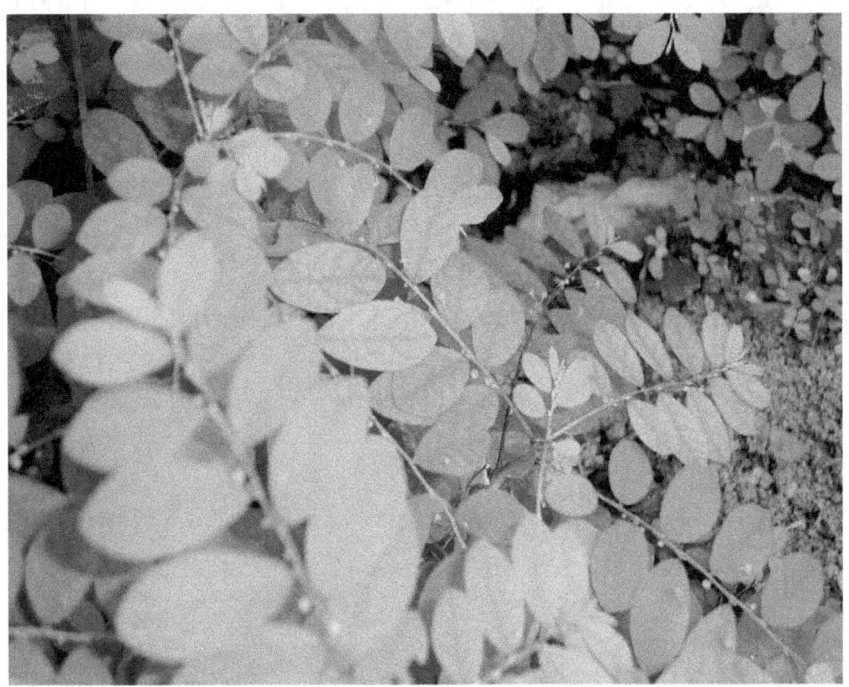

Botanical Name : Phyllanthus amarus

Other Species : Phyllanthus airy-shawii, Phyllanthus debilis, Phyllanthus fraternus, Phyllanthus niruri

Family : Euphorbiaceae

Appearance : Annual herb with closely arranged leaves. Flower-minute, yellowish green in clusters. Seeds - 6 black, triangular with longitudinal leaves.

Medicinal Parts : Whole plant, root, leaves.

Distribution : A native of America, now a circumtropical weed.

Karisilanganni

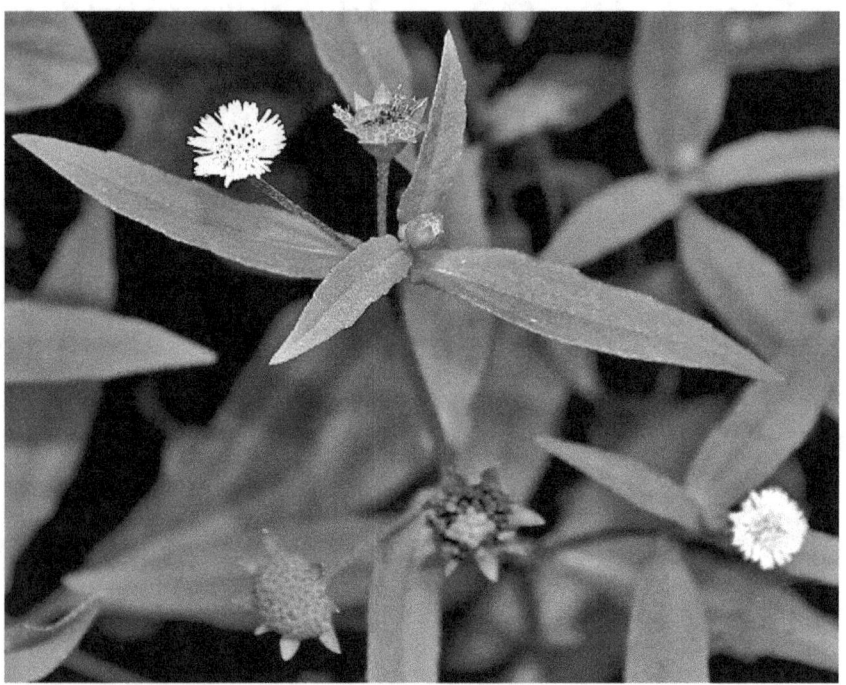

Botanical Name : Eclipta prostrata

Family : Asteraceae

Appearance : Two variety of plant - one has yellow flowers, and other white. Floral heads 6-8 mm in diameter.

Medicinal Parts : Leaf, Flower

Distribution : Found in India, China, Thailand and Brazil

Drumstick

(Moringa oleifera)

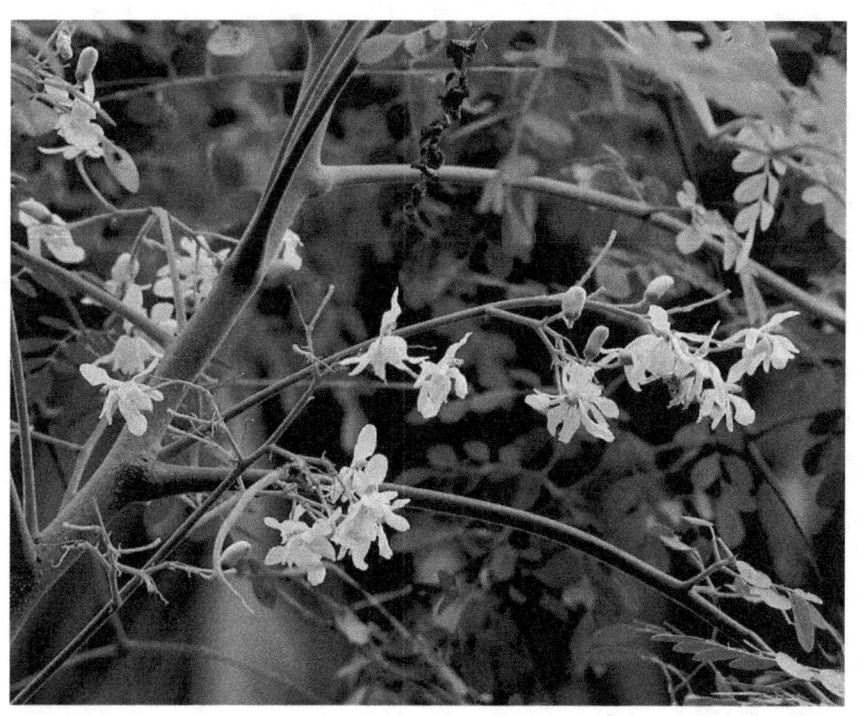

General

Because of the shape of it's fruits, the tree has come to be called 'Drumstick'. The fruits are rich in proteins, minerals, calcium, iron, phosphorous and vitamin C as well as facilitators such as folic acid which help in absorption of iron, and B-carotene, in synthesis of vitamin A. The creamy white flowers are also used in the treatment of several ailments. Its seeds, leaves and roots too find medicinal applications.

Profile

Botanical Name : Morianga oleifera

Family : Moringaceae

Appearance : A handsome tree with rough and corky bark. Leaves - fern like, divided and subdivided. Flowers - while and honey scented. Fruits - elongated, 3-angular, resembling drumsticks.

Medicinal Parts : Gum, flowers, leaves, roots, seed oil

Distribution : Common throughout India.

Preparation and Dose

Fry 1/2 tsp black pepper powder in 1 tbsp ghee. Add 2 cups fresh drumstick leaves and stir-fry for 3 minutes.

Eat with steamed rice or bread for 40 days.

Fenugreek

(Trigonella foenum-graecum)

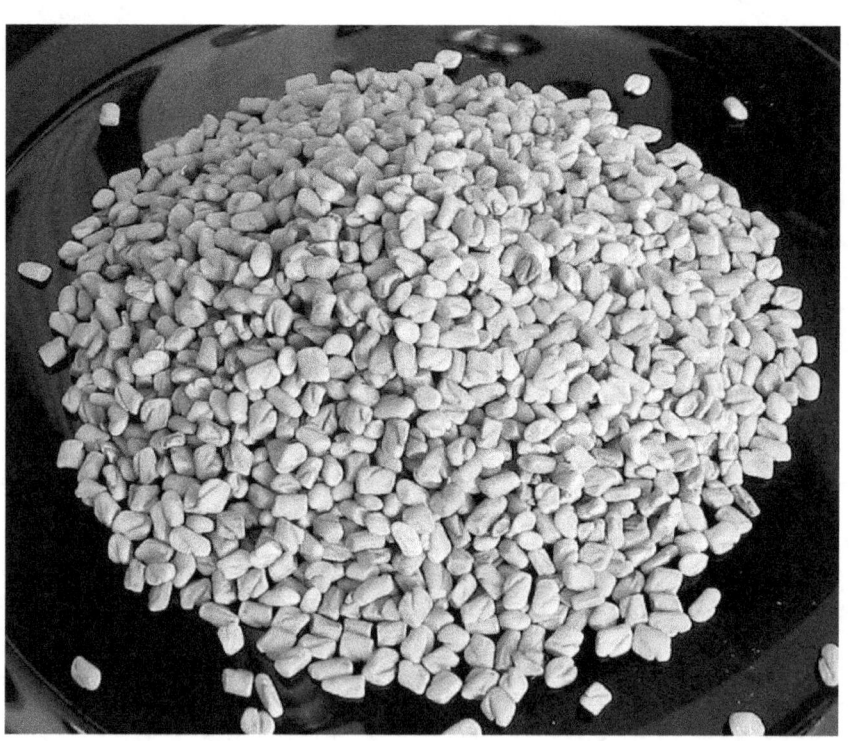

General

Fenugreek seeds are rich in iron and hence helpful in combating anaemia. It is also used to cure a number of common ailments – cough, fever, bronchitis, boils, ulcers..

Profile

Botanical Name : Trigonella foenum-graecum

Family : Leguminoseae

Appearance : Strong scented, erect, robust, annual herb with light green, pinnate, tri-foliate leaves. Flowers – yellow. Pods – beaked. Seeds – brownish yellow with peculiar odour, oblong with deep groove across one corner.

Medicinal Parts : leaves, seeds

Distribution : Cultivated worldwide as a semi-arid crop.

Preparation and Dose

2 tsp fenugreek seeds cooked with 1 cup rice. Eat with a little salt regularly for a fortnight.

Guggul

(Commiphora mukul)

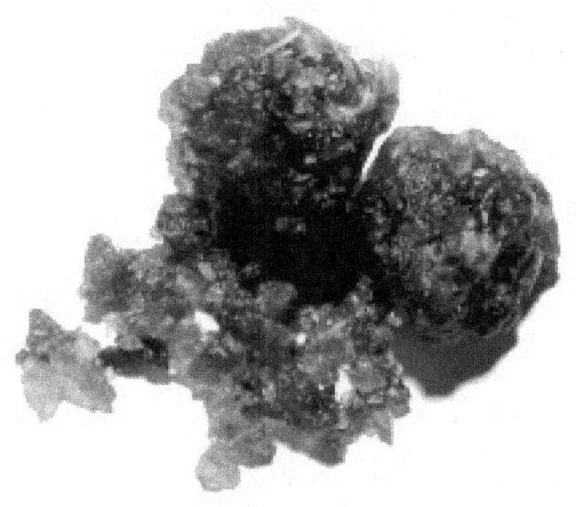

General

A shrub growing in arid, rocky wastelands with out-streched branches and sparing leaves. Guggul is the source of Indian Bdellium, a gum exuded by the plant during harsh summer months. It is dull green or brown in color with a balsamic odour and a bitter aromatic taste.

Profile

Botanical Name : Commiphora wightii, Commiphora mukul, Balsamodendron roxburghii

Other Species : Commiphora myrrha

Family : Burseraceae

Appearance : A slow growing shrub with knotty, spiny branches. Leaflets 1-3 toothed. Flowers brownish red. Fruits red. The cut surface of plant secretes a gum, which is a lustrous, pale brown, semi solid mass.

Medicinal Parts : Oleoresin (Gum)

Distribution : The guggul plant may be found from northern Africa to central Asia, but is most common in northern India. It grows wild in rocky, arid areas of Gujrat, Karnataka, and Rajasthan in India.

Preparation and Dose

Take 1/4 tsp guggul powder along with honey and lime juice on a empty stomach in the morning.

Mandukaparni

(Centella asiatica)

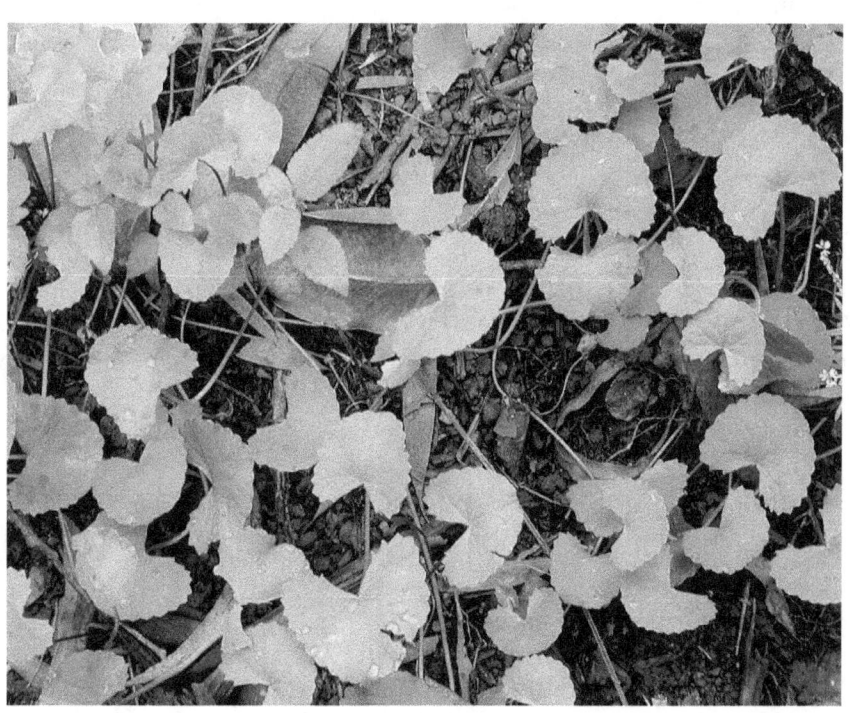

General

Mandukaparni in Sanskrit refers to shape and appearance of leaves of this plant, which resemble the webbed feet of a frog. The leaves also have a strong resemblance to human brain. The herb has been popular in the entire South East Asia besides China, Tibet, Japan and India.

Profile

Botanical Name : Centella asiatica

Other Species : Hydrocotyle asiatica

Family : Apiaceae

Appearance : A creeper bearing roots on nodes. Leaves - small, rounded/kidney shaped, with toothed margins. Flowers - pinkish red, minute, 3-6 in clusters. Fruits - small, 7-9 ridged.

Medicinal Parts : Whole plant - leaves, roots, seeds, stem

Distribution : Throughout India and SE Asia, in moist places, marshy banks of water bodies and irrigated fields.

Preparation and Dose

Mix 1/2 tsp leaf juice with 1 tsp honey and take for 30 days.

Papaya

(Carica papaya)

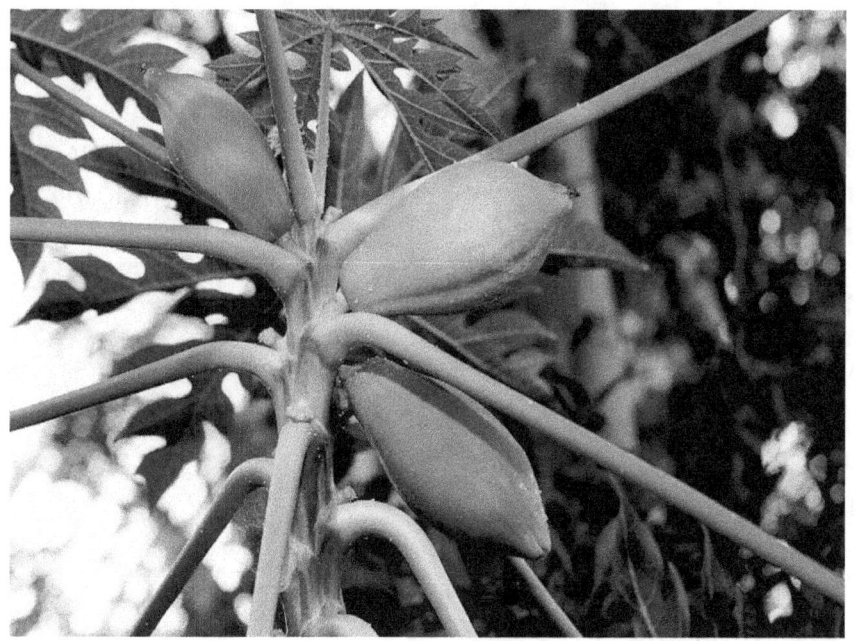

General

Nearly every inch of papaya tree possesses medicinal properties. Like the legendary apple, a papaya a day can also keep the doctor away.

Profile

Botanical Name : Carica papaya

Family : Caricaceae

Appearance : A tree having soft wood with palm like leaves. Male and female flowers are on separate trees. The fruit is large, oblong or nearly spherical fleshy berry with yellow orange rind like a gourd.

Medicinal Parts : Leaves, fruits(ripe or unripe), latex

Distribution : Originally from southern Mexico (particularly Chiapas and Veracruz), Central America, and northern South America, the papaya is now cultivated in most tropical countries.

Preparation and Dose

Eat papayas frequently.

Pomegranate

(Punica granatum)

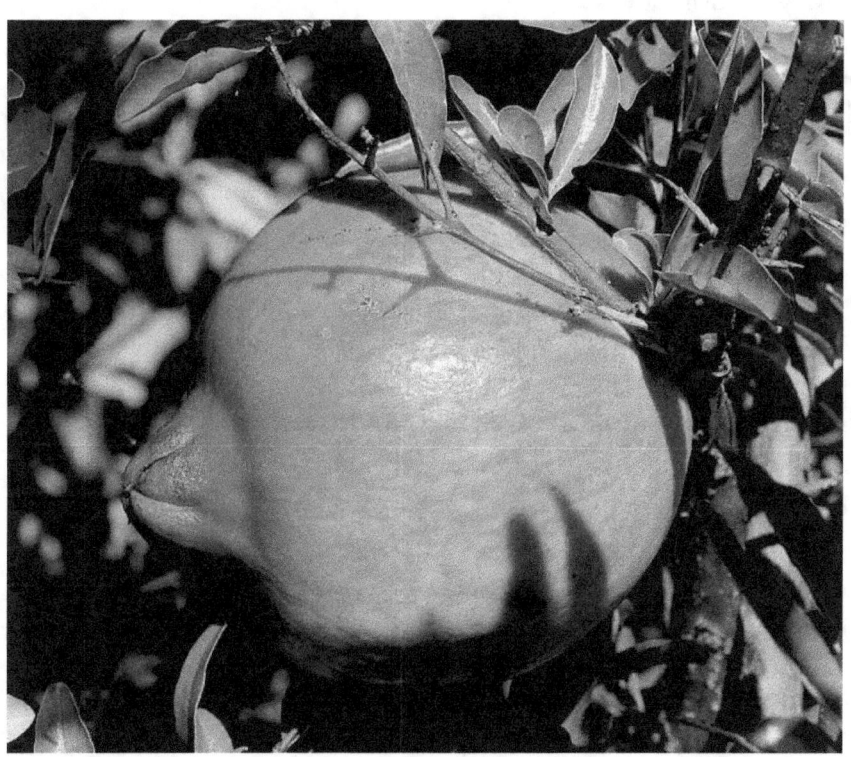

General

Growing a pomegranate tree in your garden is like having a pharmacy at your doorstep. The fruit rind has great medicinal properties. Besides the rind, flowers, stem bark and fruit also have medicinal values.

Profile

Botanical Name : Punica granatum

Family : Punicaceae

Appearance : Glabrous shrub or small tree with narrowly elliptical leaves, bright red flowers and orange-colored funnel-shaped calyx tube. Fruits – large, globose berry, yellowish red when ripe with persistent calyx lobes. Seeds – surrounded by edible, pinkish white pulp.

Medicinal Parts : Stem, stem-bark, root, seeds, buds, flowers, fruit, pulp, juice, rind, seed oil.

Distribution : Generally available in most parts of world.

Preparation and Dose

1. Grind 2-3 tsp dried seeds and take once or twice along with milk every day; or

2. Dissolve ¼ tsp cinnamon and 2 tsp honey in 1 cup pomegranate juice and drink everyday.

Rose

(Rosa centifolia)

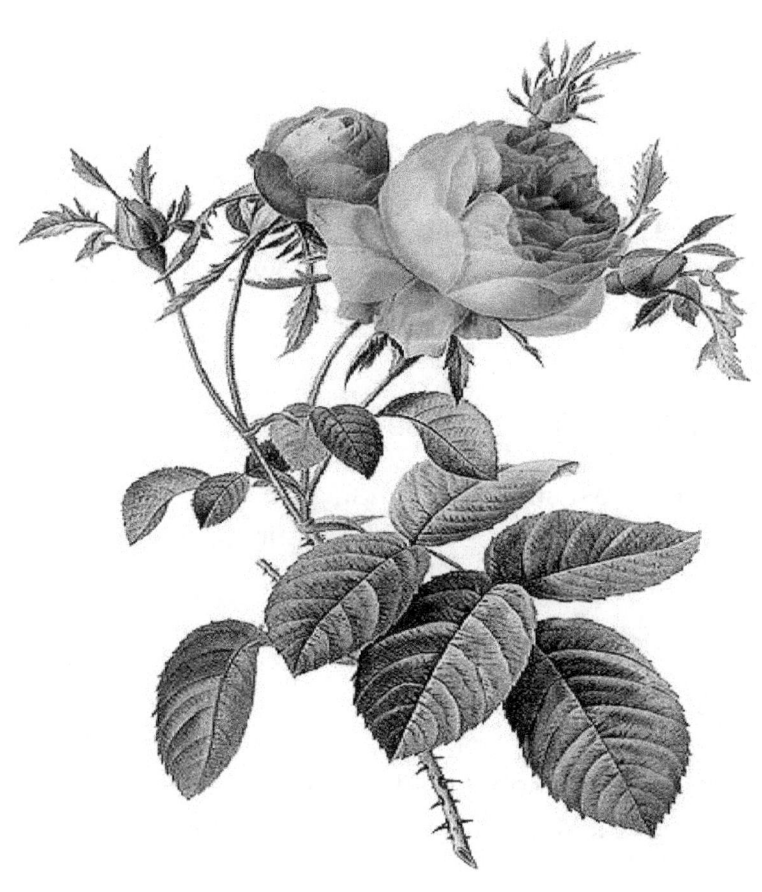

General

Rose cultivated in gardens for ornamental purposes are complex hybrids derived from many wild species. A few species are grown on a commercial scale which are used in perfumery and medicine.

Profile

Botanical Name : Rosa centifolia

Appearance : A prickly shrub, white to crimson flowers. Stems bear alternate, odd-pinnate leaves. Flowers are usually single and five petaled in wild species, but often double in cultivated varieties.

Medicinal Parts : Flowers, rose-hips

Distribution : Most species are native to Asia, with smaller numbers native to Europe, North America, and northwest Africa.

Preparation and Dose

Boil 6 tsp each crushed fennel seeds (foeniculum vulgare) and red rose petals in 1 cup water. Strain and drink twice daily.

Saunf (Fennel)

(Foeniculum vulgare)

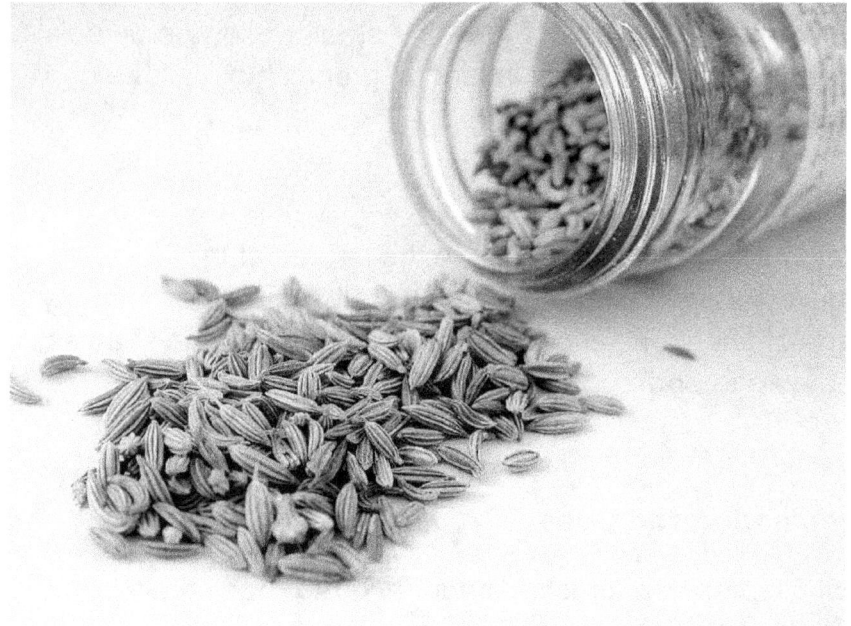

General

Saunf consists of the fruits of fennel, often wrongly called seeds. It constitutes an excellent remedy for a number of ailments.

Profile

Botanical Name : Foeniculum vulgare, Foeniculum officinale, Foeniculum capillaceum, Anethum foeniculum

Other Species : Fennel, Indian sweet fennel.

Family : Apiaceae (Formerly Umbelliferae)

Appearance : A tall glabrous aromatic herb. Leaves – pinnately decompound. Flowers – small, yellow, in umbels. Fruit – ellipsoid, 6-7 mm in length, greenish or yellowish brown.

Medicinal Parts : Roots, fruits(seeds)

Distribution : It is indigenous to the shores of the Mediterranean but has become widely naturalized in many parts of the world, especially on dry soils near the sea-coast and on riverbanks.

Preparation and Dose

Boil 6 tsp each of crushed saunf and red rose petals in 1½ teacup water and strain. Take twice daily.

Turmeric

(Curcuma longa)

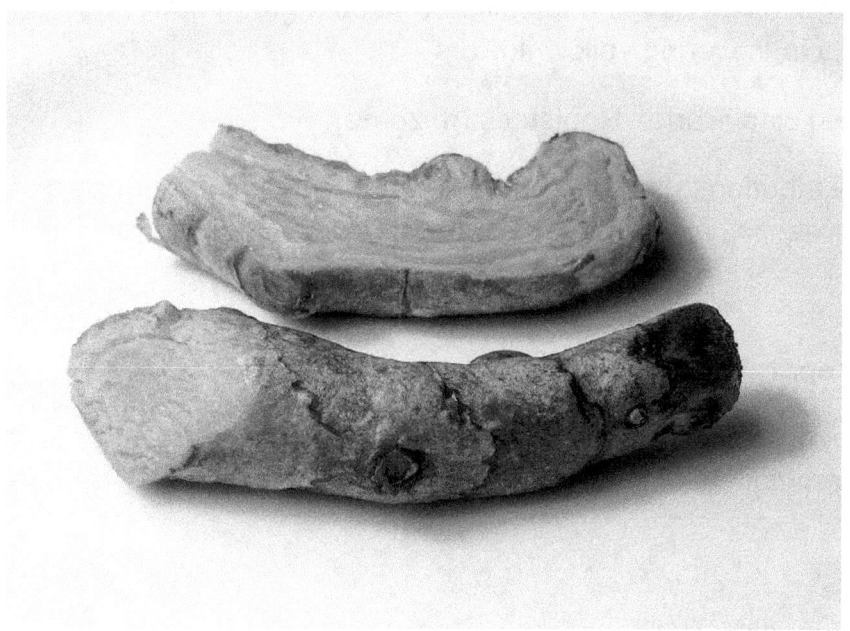

General

The turmeric which is available commercially for cooking purposes is the boiled, debarked rootstock which has lost many of its miraculous medicinal properties. The raw, dried rootstock of the plant should therefore be preferred.

Profile

Botanical Name : Curcuma longa, Curcuma domestica

Family : Zingiberaceae

Appearance : The spice turmeric consists of dried, boiled, cleaned, and polished rootstock of the plant. The plant has a large tuft of leaves and spikes with pale green flowering bracts, covering yellow flowers.

Medicinal Parts : Rootstock (rhizome)

Distribution : India and Pakistan are significant producers of turmeric.

Preparation and Dose

Take 1 tsp raw turmeric juice and honey mixed together every morning.

<u>Vasaka</u>

(Adhatoda vasica)

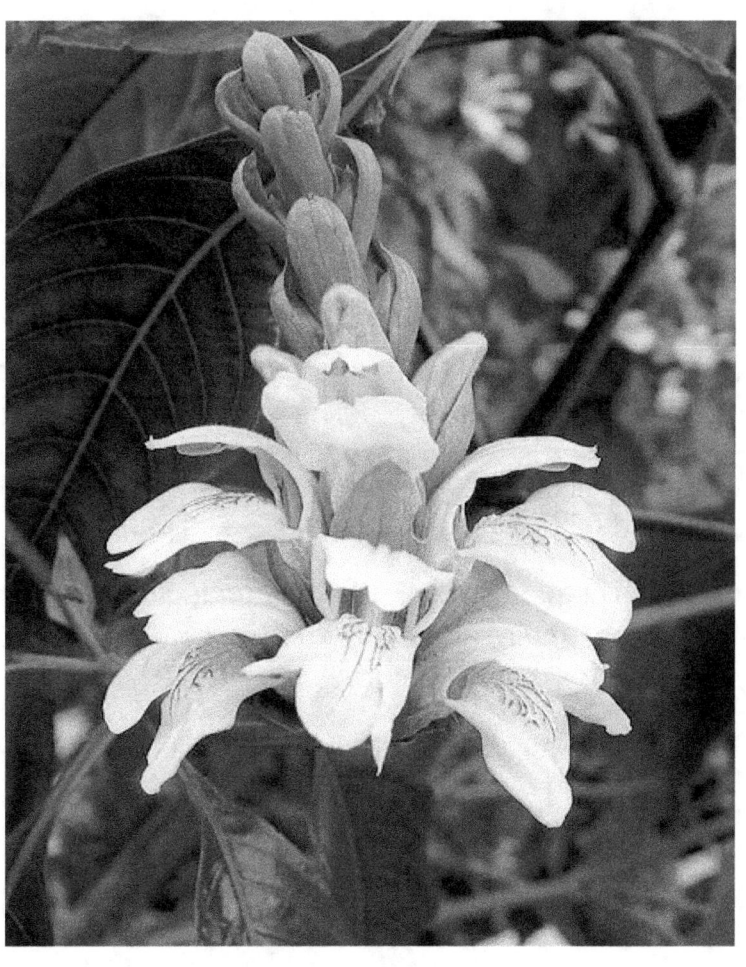

General

Vasaka grows in abundance in the lower reaches of the Himalayas. Sometimes it is cultivated as a hedge plant. The drug vasaka comes from fresh or dried leaves of the plant, and is administered in form of juice, syrup or decoction.

Profile

Botanical Name : Adhatoda vasica

Other Species : Adhatoda zeylanica, Justicia adhatoda

Family : Acanthaceae

Appearance : Tall, dense, ever green shrub. Leaves - large, lance shaped, somewhat resembling mango leaves. Fruit - a capsule with 4 seeds. Flowers - white or purple.

Medicinal Parts : Flowers, leaves, roots, and bark

Distribution : The plant grows wild in abundance all over SriLanka, Nepal, India, and the Pothohar region of Pakistan, particularly in the Pharwala area.

Preparation and Dose

Crush 1 tbsp of leaves and boil in 2 cups of water till reduced to 1 cup. Add 1 tsp honey.

Drink 1/2 cup twice a day for 40 days.

<u>Some Important Notes</u>

1. Preparation

When the herb is extremely bitter, sour, astrigent or in powdered form, it can be mixed with honey, jaggery, sugar, candy etc.

2. Dosage

The quantity of dose can vary from one person to another based on individual age, physical build, and reaction of patient to a particular formulation.

The dosage prescribed in this book is meant for fully grown and mature patients. The dose should be increased/decreased for each patient keeping in mind individual patient's constitution.

3. Effectiveness

The contents of a herbal plant part varies widely due to factors such as climate, altitude, latitude, soil type, nutrition, temperature, relative humidity, time of plucking, packaging, storage etc. Hence the effectiveness of herb for treating an ailment may vary in different cases.

Patient needs to keep in mind this inherent weakness of herbal effectiveness, and be prepared to continue the treatment for a little longer time.

Other Books That May Interest You

Herbs That Cure:

Asthma
Bad Breath
Bronchitis
Constipation
Diabetes
Diarrhoea
Fatigue
Flatulence
Genito-urinal disorders
Haemorrhoids
Hair Loss
Heart Problems
Insomnia
Joints Pain
Leucoderma
Obesity
Pimples
Psoriasis
Rheumatism
Sexual Debility
Skin Diseases
Stomach Disorders
Toothache
Venereal Diseases
Wrinkles

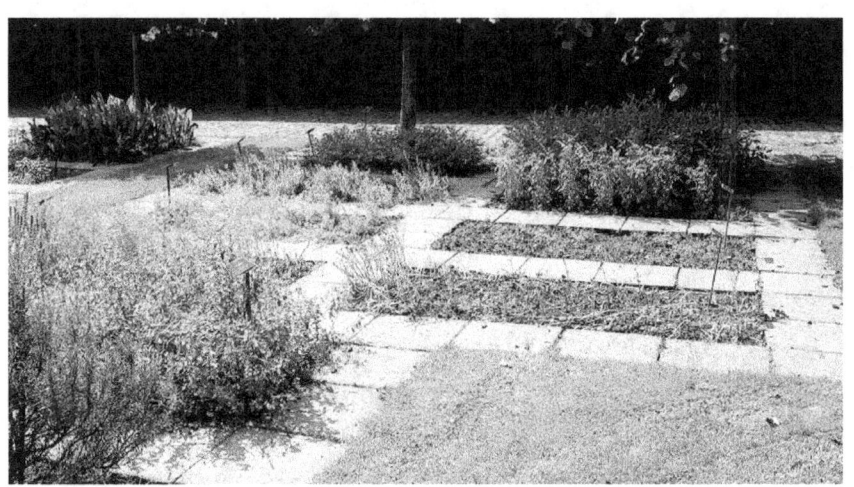